SHIATSU

MADE SIMPLE

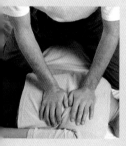
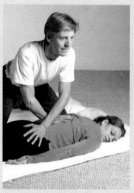
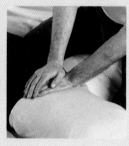

CHRIS JARMEY

Haldane **Mason**

First published in the UK in 2001 by
Haldane Mason Ltd
59 Chepstow Road
London W2 5BP
email: haldane.mason@pipex.com

ISBN 1-902463-50-1

A Haldane Mason Book

Editors: Kate Latham, Elizabeth Rowe
Designer: Rachel Clark
Photographer: Sue Ford
Models: Victoria Caswell, George Dellar, Cristiane Guida de Camargo, Terrence Hill, Chris Jarmey

Colour reproduction by CK Litho Ltd, UK

Printed in China

Important

The information in this book is generally applicable but is not tailored to specific circumstances or individuals. The author and publishers can accept no responsibility for any problems arising from following the information given in this book. Safety information is supplied on page 7 which should be read before attempting to practise shiatsu. If in doubt about any of the techniques described, please consult your doctor or an experienced shiatsu practitioner.

Contents

Introduction   4

How Shiatsu Works   8

How to apply Shiatsu Technique   16

Do-in Exercises   36

Simple Sequence in the   42
Prone Position

Simple Sequence in the   52
Side Position

Useful Contacts   62

Index   64

Introduction

Shiatsu is a Japanese word which, literally translated, means 'finger pressure'. However, shiatsu is much more than that. Its techniques involve the use not only of the fingers, but also of the thumbs, palms, knees, forearms, elbows and feet. Since shiatsu is given on the floor rather than on a bed, it places considerable emphasis on the correct positioning of the body and makes extensive use of gravity.

Shiatsu is a physical therapy which is applied at floor level with the minimum amount of physical effort on the part of the therapist, and which uses oriental medicine as its theoretical framework. To reach a professional standard of competence generally takes at least three years of committed study and practice.

Beyond its role in the healing of others, shiatsu is also of tremendous importance in self-development. It focuses the mind and grounds both body and mind in much the same way as Tai Ji Quan (sometimes spelt Tai Chi Chuan), yoga and various forms of meditation.

A brief history of shiatsu

Although the word 'shiatsu' was not coined until the early 20th century, the roots of the therapy lie firmly within traditional oriental medicine and a system of self-massage and self-applied pressure point therapy known as Do-In (Japanese) or Dao-Yinn (Chinese). Do-in gradually spread from China into south-east Asia and then into Korea.

By the 10th century AD, Chinese medicine had been introduced into Japan. There, an amalgam of palm healing, acupressure and massage, known collectively as Anma, combined with Do-in to form a practice which loosely resembled present-day shiatsu.

Around 300 years ago, Japanese doctors were required to study Anma as a means of familiarizing themselves with the human structure, energy channels and pressure points. Anma helped them to diagnose disease accurately and to choose the most appropriate treatment for patients, whether it was acupuncture, herbal medicine or bodywork. Gradually, however, Anma was reduced to treating simple muscular tensions until, by the 20th century, it was licensed only to promote pleasure and comfort.

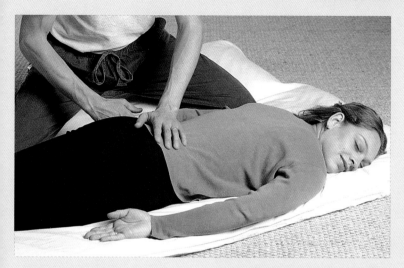

However, there were still many Anma therapists who based their work on the original theory. They coined the name shiatsu in order to avoid the restrictive regulations applied to Anma. The Japanese government eventually recognized shiatsu as a legitimate form of therapy in the mid-1950s.

Shiatsu did not become widely known in Europe and the United States until the 1970s, although it has been practised by a few Japanese and Occidentals in the West since its conception.

The giver can only realize the full potential of shiatsu after he or she has developed certain qualities:

• The ability to remain relaxed and comfortable at any given time, irrespective of which technique is being used.

• The ability to detect subtle changes in a person's vitality through touch.

• The ability to assess a person's state of health through the development of a greater empathy and the understanding of oriental medicine.

The shiatsu environment

All that is required for shiatsu is a floor area large enough for the receiver's thin futon. There should be enough space around it for the practitioner to move about. A futon of two to three layers is ideal, preferably wide enough to allow the practitioner's knees some cushioning when practising.

Shiatsu is better done through clothing, since working on the skin stimulates too many superficial sensory nerves, thus distracting the receiver from experiencing deeper sensations. The practitioner can also feel for deeper levels of imbalance in the body when the sensation of skin-to-skin contact is removed.

Ideally, the recipient should wear a single layer of loose-fitting, cotton garments (natural fibres allow a more effective shiatsu connection).

The 'tools' of shiatsu

The primary tools for giving shiatsu are the palms, thumbs and fingers. Depending on which treatment strategy is adopted, the therapist will use his thumbs or fingertips if he needs to apply very specific pressure to a pressure point.

To work on a more generalized area, he is more likely to use his palms. If particularly strong pressure is needed, then the forearms, elbows, knees or feet may be used.

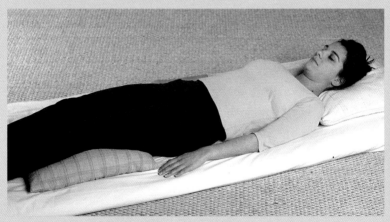

Ensure that the receiver is comfortable and relaxed before treatment begins.

Cautionary guidelines

This book is for beginners, and meant only as a supplement to personal or class instruction from an experienced shiatsu teacher. You should practise the techniques it contains only on people who are fit and well.

Your shiatsu mantra should be 'if in doubt, don't do it'. If you attend shiatsu classes, you will learn if and when you can and cannot give shiatsu to people with certain problems. You should not try to learn purely from a book. You cannot ask a book questions and a book cannot oversee your technique or correct your attitude.

Do not work directly on painful areas, such as tight or pulled muscles, ligament injuries or joint tenderness. It should be possible to work around these areas instead.

In addition, you should avoid giving shiatsu to women during their first three months of pregnancy. For the remainder of the pregnancy, you should avoid giving shiatsu below the knee (i.e. avoid the lower leg and foot). This is because there are several pressure points or *tsubos* in this area which can initiate a miscarriage.

Advice for the practitioner

As a beginner, you should not practise shiatsu on people who are suffering from:
- arthritis
- rheumatoid arthritis
- high or low blood pressure
- contagious diseases
- fever
- cancer
- heart disease
- life-threatening conditions.

You should also avoid those parts of the receiver's body affected by:
- varicose veins
- burns
- open sores
- broken bones
- bruises.

How *Shiatsu* Works

Shiatsu is based on traditional oriental medicine and the concept that a series of energy channels runs through the body and determines its state of health. This section will explain the basic principles, concentrating on *tsubos* or pressure points, the flow of ki energy through the body, and how blockages of ki can be cleared and deficiencies corrected.

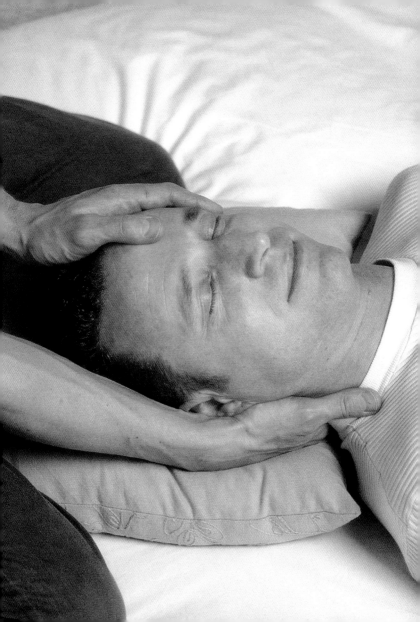

What is shiatsu?

Shiatsu is based on the concept that applying specific physical manipulation techniques to particular areas of your body will improve your overall health. The manner in which shiatsu is applied determines its precise effect.

There are three broad categories of shiatsu technique:

Tonification
Where sustained pressure is applied at the optimum angle to reach deep into the *tsubos* or pressure points. This will increase the level of energy and blood circulating through a particular area.

Dispersal
Active techniques, such as shaking, rocking, stretching, circling and squeezing, disperse blocked or engorged energy and blood. This is also called 'sedation'.

Calming
Light, stationary holding with the palm, using minimal or no pressure, or very gentle rocking, will calm agitated energy.

A shiatsu session will generally include all three of these methods, with a particular emphasis on one depending on the predominant type of energy imbalance.

During all tonification techniques, most calming techniques and many dispersal techniques, one hand actively applies the technique while the palm of the other hand feels for reactions elsewhere in the body.

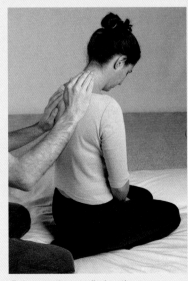

Palm cupping applied to the upper back is a dispersal technique.

Channels and the circulation of ki

The theory behind shiatsu lies in traditional oriental philosophy and medicine, which considers everything in nature to be a manifestation of energy. This universal energy is called ki (sometimes spelt qi or ch'i). Ki links all the functions and organs of the body together through a system of interconnecting channels (sometimes called meridians) which are shown in the diagram on page 12. The basic channels are the same as those used in acupuncture, although there are some extensions to these channels in shiatsu.

A ki channel flows partly inside the body, to connect with the organs, and partly near the surface of the body. It is those channel sections near the surface of the body which are accessible to shiatsu. All the ki channels are connected to each other to form a continuous flow, animating all parts of the body as it passes through. The aim of shiatsu is to keep the ki flowing evenly.

Many channels have been identified, fourteen of which contain pressure points that influence the organs and associated bodily functions. Twelve of the channels are named after the organ through which they pass – for example, the kidney channel, the bladder channel, the liver channel and so on.

The body and mind are not mutually exclusive. By affecting the body, we can affect the mind, and vice versa. According to oriental medicine, each channel corresponds to aspects of the mind and emotions, as well as physical areas of the body. For example, the channel which runs through the kidneys influences willpower, drive and the capacity for fear. It is also a major factor in the growth and strength of bones, nerves and brain tissue, and it also influences the balance of water and minerals within the body.

In shiatsu terminology, a fullness or blockage of ki in a channel or pressure point is referred to as 'jitsu', whereas a weakness or emptiness of ki is known as 'kyo'. The aim of shiatsu is to discover the root cause behind any acute or chronic disharmony and to attempt to stabilize it via the tonification of the kyo or the dispersal of the jitsu within the channels. Jitsu areas are easy to find because they feel active and may protrude from the surface. Kyo areas are more difficult to locate because they exhibit little reaction, and are hidden below the surface. Sensitive shiatsu, done all over the body, will highlight these kyo/jitsu divergences and re-harmonize the general level and flow of ki.

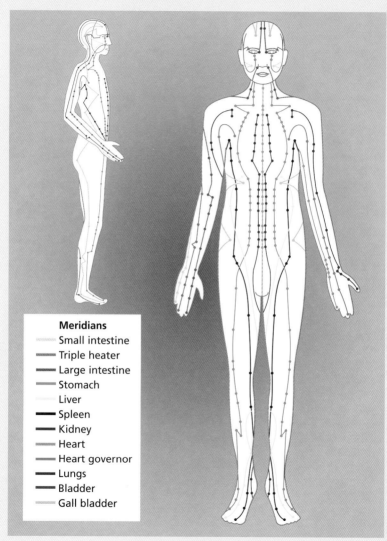

Meridians
- Small intestine
- Triple heater
- Large intestine
- Stomach
- Liver
- Spleen
- Kidney
- Heart
- Heart governor
- Lungs
- Bladder
- Gall bladder

The twelve organ meridians, with tsubos *marked as dots on each channel.*

A good professional shiatsu practitioner will be able to assess which channels are most lacking in ki, and which are blocked. If the blockages are balanced against the deficiencies, the imbalances in the other channels will also be reduced.

The concept and 'structure' of a *tsubo*

At specific locations along the ki channels, there are 'gateways' or 'cavities' where ki can be accessed from the surface. These gateways are known as *tsubos* (pressure points). A *tsubo* looks like a vase-shaped swirl of energy with a wide mouth leading into a narrower neck, which then widens into a broad belly.

Each of the primary channels has a number of 'fixed' *tsubos*. After many years of documented observation, each *tsubo* now has a name and a number and a record of its action on the body and mind when stimulated.

As well as the fixed *tsubos*, there are a number of 'transient' *tsubos* which come and go along the channels between the 'fixed' *tsubos*. They arise where and when they do because there is either a lack of ki or an excessive build-up of ki in that place and at that point in time.

Where the ki is lacking, the *tsubo* will feel lifeless and empty, lacking vitality and elasticity. Where the ki

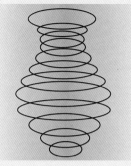

A tsubo is a vortex of ki energy.

is blocked and consequently overcrowded, there will be a feeling of fullness, tightness and constriction and that place will often be painful to the touch.

Shiatsu is a method of bodywork which aims to re-balance the activity of ki in and around the *tsubos*.

Tsubo points and ki energy
Tsubos are essentially points where ki can:
• access the channel from outside the body
• leave the channel to connect with the outside world
• represent distortions in the channel flow, so that, when activated (by pressure, for example), the ki can affect the channel and therefore some aspect of the body/mind function.

Shiatsu and the autonomic nervous system

Shiatsu therapy draws upon an extensive theoretical base and range of practical approaches, and can offer an almost endless selection of techniques. However, a correctly applied shiatsu session consisting only of the basic techniques, without working specifically on the channels and without using the tools of diagnosis and oriental medicine theory, will still have a tremendously positive effect upon the receiver.

In a nutshell, shiatsu at any level is incredibly relaxing, revitalizing and it also strengthens the immune system. Why? Because it invokes the para-sympathetic response of the autonomic nervous system (ANS), which, in simple English, means it causes a deep relaxation response.

Rather than get heavily into the physiology of the ANS, all you need to know is that we have physiological and psychological responses to threat which are very different from our reactions to safe and supportive situations.

When we are under threat, we become very alert to enable us to assess the gravity and detail of the situation rapidly and thus give ourselves the best chance of counteracting or escaping from whatever it is that is threatening us. Depending on the level of threat, we may be required to defend ourselves, either by fighting it out or by running away.

When under threat, our bodies automatically send more adrenaline into the blood and more blood to the muscles, ensuring their optimum performance. Our breathing rhythm accelerates to enable enough oxygen to get to our muscles and brain, and our senses of hearing, seeing and smelling grow more acute. We become 'ready for action'.

By contrast, when we feel safe and not under pressure, we tend to 'let go' and relax. Our breathing slows down and our eyes and ears become less sharply focused.

If you touch someone in the correct way, at the appropriate time and with the right attitude, the touch will soothe and support them. You have probably experienced a hand on your shoulder from the right person at the right time when you were upset. It helped, didn't it? Conversely, that shove from someone who saw you as being 'in the way' certainly did not make you feel good. I bet you felt irritated, and your muscles tensed up.

So, if you push someone, you can expect them to tense up and assume a closed, defensive posture, or even an aggressive stance towards you. If you offer a supportive contact, such as catching someone when they trip, their attitude to you is likely to be positive and this will be reflected in a reduction of their bodily tensions when interacting with you. Try leaning against a good friend when you are tired; they will instinctively support you. Then push them and see what happens!

Shiatsu technique emphasizes this leaning, 'humanizing' principle. You always lean, rather than push, to apply pressure. In other words, pressure is applied using your body weight rather than your muscular strength.

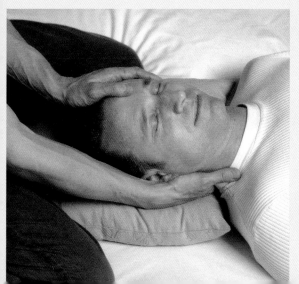

Shiatsu encourages a deep relaxation response, achieved by leaning and relaxing, rather than by pushing and shoving.

How
to apply
Shiatsu
Technique

The fingertips are the basic tools for applying shiatsu, although elbows, forearms, thumbs and knees may also be used depending on the particular method. The following section shows you the correct posture for practising shiatsu and techniques using a range of shiatsu 'tools'.

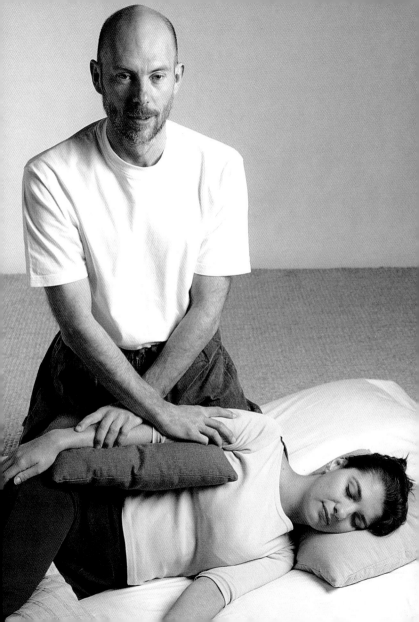

Position and posture

Shiatsu technique should never come from muscular strength, but should use gravity wherever possible. That is, one should lean rather than push or pull. To lean correctly, you need to be aware of your centre of gravity, which is your belly, or *hara*, as it is called in Japanese (and therefore in shiatsu). If you ensure that your movements originate from your *hara*, then they will involve your whole body, thereby utilizing all your body's power.

To be more specific, all movement should originate from a point just below the navel, which is your central pivotal point. This point is known as the tanden; the focal point of the *hara*.

Watch a baby move and it is very clear that its movements originate from its centre, the belly. You never see young babies tensing their shoulders to push a toy. If you can persuade a baby to crawl on your back, you will experience the key qualities of shiatsu contact: the complete surrender of weight to gravity, with both movements and balance centred and emanating from the belly.

How to position your body in relation to the receiver

When giving shiatsu, it is important to make sure that your *hara* is aligned with the area upon which you are working; or to get as close

to that ideal as is practical, without sacrificing your comfort. In other words, the more you relax your body when applying pressure, the more you can use your body weight.

If your *hara* is aligned with your direction of pressure, your ki will connect with the receiver to a greater degree. Connecting your ki simply means aligning your intention with your action or, in other words, taking the most direct route to reach your goal.

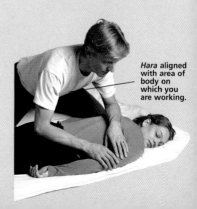

Hara aligned with area of body on which you are working.

The correct posture for giving shiatsu

It is important to hold yourself correctly while giving shiatsu. Correct posture will make it easier for you to support the receiver's body without getting tired. In addition, it will enable you to move around their body more efficiently and generally help your ki to flow smoothly.

The basic rules of good shiatsu posture are:
- adopt a wide base with your legs, to ensure a low centre of gravity
- keep your *hara* relaxed and open
- look ahead, not down at the receiver (but check occasionally to make sure they are comfortable)
- keep your shoulders relaxed
- keep your chest open
- keep the back of your neck open, lengthened and relaxed. Imagine that the spaces within the joints of your spine, shoulder, elbows, wrist and fingers are constantly opening as they relax more.

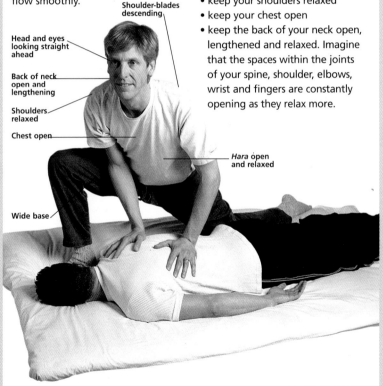

Shoulder-blades descending

Head and eyes looking straight ahead

Back of neck open and lengthening

Shoulders relaxed

Chest open

Hara open and relaxed

Wide base

Using palms

No special equipment is required to give shiatsu. The only 'tools' you need to apply the techniques are the different parts of your body. The part you use depends upon the type of connection and pressure you wish to give. When you are a beginner, open palms, thumbs, forearms and knees are the predominant tools. Experienced practitioners will sometimes apply specialized techniques.

The palms are the main tools used in beginner-level shiatsu. Although less specific in their use than thumbs

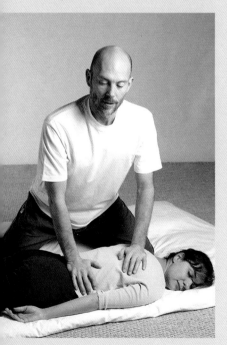

or fingertips, the palms have a more soothing quality. If a friend is distressed, we are naturally inclined to place a palm on his or her shoulder as a gesture of support, rather than lean a thumb into their back! Also, the palms are icons of interpersonal communication, as illustrated by the gesture of shaking the hand of someone you meet.

When practising palm techniques, the whole surface of your palm should be kept in full contact with the recipient so that you can mould your hand around the contours of their body. Your palms will therefore lie flat on their back, or curl to envelop an arm or an ankle. The palms and fingers must remain relaxed. The arms should remain outstretched, but with the elbows unlocked.

Arms are outstretched, without tensing the muscles, and elbows are unlocked.

For closer body contact, it may be necessary to have your arms bent at the elbow at an angle of 90º, with the knee or inner thigh supporting your upper arm. However, this will cause a slight reduction in the connection of ki flow between your *hara* and your palm.

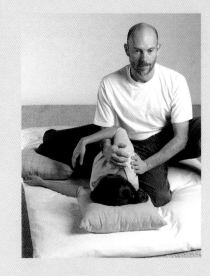

Elbows are bent and supported by the knee or inner thigh. This can be useful for a side position technique.

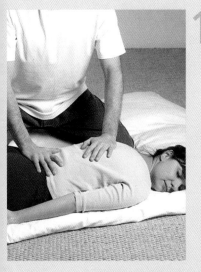

Support hand technique

Keep both hands apart, but in contact with the receiver. This is the most basic yet most important therapeutic shiatsu technique. It enables us to 'listen' with one hand, while the other hand is used to tonify, calm or disperse ki. The 'listening' hand (the practitioner's left hand in the photograph) is often called the support hand or the mother hand. The active hand is sometimes called the working hand or the child hand.

When tonifying, the working hand should be applied at right angles to the area of contact.

21

2 Palm overlap technique

Place one hand on top of the other. This technique can be used when a malleable, wave-like action is required. It is often used directly on the receiver's belly to ease congestion or constipation.

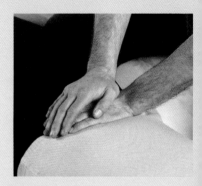

3 Circular rotations

With one palm moulded into the contours of the shoulder blade, buttocks or sacrum, firmly rotate the connective tissues over the underlying bone. The other palm can be positioned either nearby on the body, or on top of the working hand.

4 Grasping

One hand clasps the limb for support, while the other moves along the limb. Alternatively, both hands can clasp a limb as you stretch that limb away from the space between your hands.

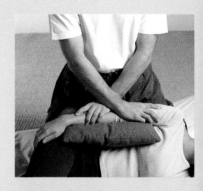

Double palm squeezing

Interlock your fingers and apply a squeezing movement simultaneously with the heels of both hands. This method is useful for squeezing the muscles on either side of the lumbar spine, from the kidney region down to the pelvis.

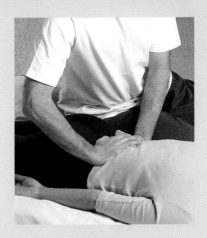

Palm off the body technique

Holding the palms slightly away from the body has a warming effect if the giver is relaxed and centred. This method is especially effective when applied over the face, which can be a nice way to conclude a session. When ki sensitivity is developed, any local excess or deficiency of ki can be clearly assessed using this technique.

Using thumbs

The thumb is the classic tool of shiatsu. Some styles of shiatsu use the thumb almost exclusively, although this severely limits the potential of this therapy. One tool is rarely enough to treat a range of variable situations.

The thumb is shorter and thicker than the other fingers, having only one interphalangeal joint instead of two. This makes it the strongest individual digit and capable of applying and sustaining powerful pressure if necessary.

The ball of the thumb is used for most applications, although the area near the tip can be employed when working with light pressure between small muscle groups such as those in the neck.

Some people have very flexible thumbs that bend backwards when pressure is applied through them. If your thumb is of this type you run the risk of overstraining the interphalangeal joint and should minimize the use of your thumbs. Instead, you should make more use of your palms or fingers.

You may have difficulty keeping your thumbs straight and find that they buckle at the interphalangeal joint. If you continue to apply strong pressure like this over a period of time, you will damage your thumb

joints. Even light pressure given with buckled thumbs is discouraged. This is because ki moves in straight lines or smooth curves. Ki does not make sharp, right-angled turns. Therefore, if your thumbs are buckled, you will feel less and give less through them.

There are two main methods for supporting your thumb when applying pressure; the open hand and the closed hand methods.

1 Open hand technique

For maximum stability, it is preferable to have your thumb in contact with the receiver's body and your other four fingers spread lightly in contact.

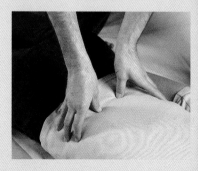

Closed hand technique

Alternatively, the four fingers can be formed into a fist so that the thumb is supported against the index finger.

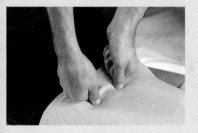

The next two methods of thumb application – the Thumb adjacent technique and the Thumb overlap technique – enable more pressure to be applied. However, such heavy pressure is unnecessary if your awareness is accurately focused.

Thumb adjacent technique

The thumbs are placed side by side, either in an open hand or closed hand configuration.

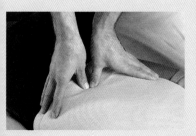

Thumb overlap technique

One thumb is placed directly on top of the other. The weight is given mostly through the top thumb, allowing the lower thumb to be more passive. Again, the open or closed hand method can be used for support.

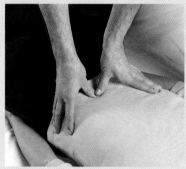

Thumb overlap technique with open hand support.

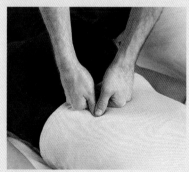

Thumb overlap technique with closed hand support.

Using fingers

The fingertips are excellent tools for sensing the ki within the channels and feeling other subtle activity registering near the surface of the receiver's body. This is because the fingers have a rich supply of sensory nerve endings. Do make sure you keep your fingernails and thumbnails short. Fingernails have no sensory nerve endings, so you will feel nothing through them. However, the receiver will certainly feel something if you dig your fingernails into them!

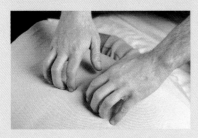

1 Three/four-finger technique

Using the middle three fingers simultaneously is a good method for tracking along a ki channel to find the discrepancies of ki within it.

Alternatively, placing all four fingers of one hand on the receiver's mid or upper back and circling or shaking them can be an effective way to disperse tension in the intercostal muscles between the ribs.

A two-handed version of the latter technique can be used to disperse any tension in the muscles close to the spine, using a push-pull movement known as *kenbiki*.

Your thumbs should be relaxed and your fingers strong (constant practice will quickly strengthen them). Like all shiatsu techniques, the movement must originate from your *hara*, with a sense of connection to your *tanden*. This will prevent fatigue and tension accumulating in your wrists.

2 Index finger technique

This technique is particularly useful for applying pressure to the side of the nose.

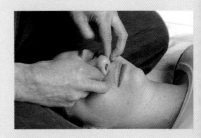

26

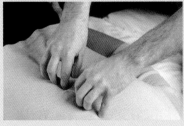

Dispersing claw technique

The thumb and fingers are slightly curled to form a claw. The claw is then pressed into the body and quickly withdrawn, as if pulling strands out of the body. In reality, excess ki is being pulled out of the area that is being worked on.

Tonifying claw technique

Similar to the Dispersing claw technique, with fingers and thumbs held closer together. Thumbs are kept straight and the fingers only slightly curved. This technique is particularly good for working down both sides of the spine at the same time.

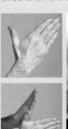
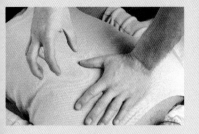

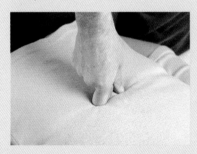

Dragon's mouth technique

Spread your thumb and index finger wide. Contact is applied through the wide-angle 'V' shape, created using one or two hands. The method is used primarily to apply pressure to the occiput (the back of the neck), and to the limbs with fingers bent.

Baby dragon's mouth

Make a fist, but with your thumb and index finger in an open 'V' shape. Like the Tonifying claw technique, this is used mainly for working down both sides of the spine at once, in the sitting, side and face-down positions.

Other hand techniques

Other hand techniques are occasionally used to disperse ki blockages, as well as to increase blood and lymph supply to the skin and the superficial muscles.

These techniques have a very localized effect and are therefore subsidiary to the mainstream shiatsu techniques and sequences featured in this book.

Used by themselves, they are fairly superficial in effect. Even so, beginners should not apply these techniques to a chronically ill person, because the receiver will be weakened still further if his or her ki is dispersed too much. Therefore, except in particular circumstances, these techniques are best kept as useful adjuncts for loosening up robust and healthy recipients, especially in the sitting or prone positions.

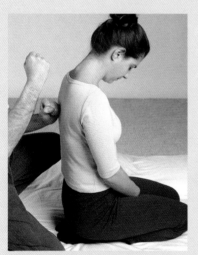

1 Pummelling with loose fists applied to receiver in sitting position.

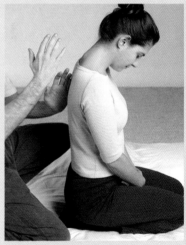

2 Loose finger chopping applied to receiver in sitting position.

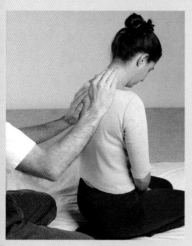

Palm cupping applied to receiver in sitting position.

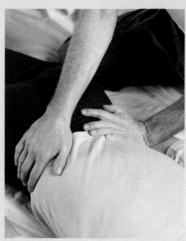

Rocking applied to receiver in prone position.

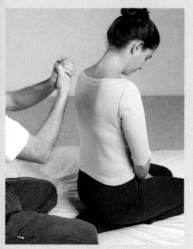

Double hand cushioning applied to receiver in sitting position.

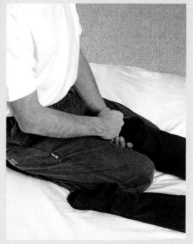

Knuckle rolling applied to receiver's feet in prone position.

Using forearms, elbows, knees and feet

Although hands are the main shiatsu tools, other limbs can be used for a range of shiatsu techniques on all areas of the body for a stronger or more specific effect.

Using forearms

The area of your forearm close to your elbow can be used to apply strong pressure to the back, hips and feet. The forearm, or both forearms together, should be used only after the area to be worked on has been manipulated by the hands. This is because your forearms are far less sensitive than your hands. One forearm applied to the sole of the foot gives a great feeling of 'ironing-out' tension. Make sure your wrist is totally relaxed.

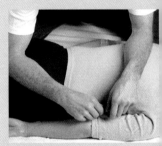

Use both forearms together on the back, buttocks or thighs to stretch the area.

Using elbows

The elbows can be used on the same areas of the body as the forearms, when a stronger and more focused pressure is required. An acutely flexed elbow gives the strongest pressure, which in most cases is too strong. An open elbow joint angle gives a more comfortable pressure. It is essential to keep the wrist relaxed and the fist open.

You should not use your elbow until you have developed a high level of sensitivity with your other 'tools', such as your palms.

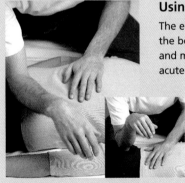

Elbow applied to back with an open angle, and with an acute angle (inset).

30

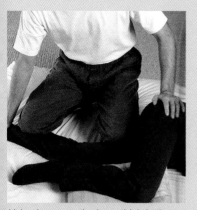

Using knees on the inner thigh in the side position.

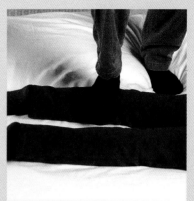

Shaking of foot on calf muscles. Avoid the knee joint.

Using knees

You can give very firm pressure with your knees but, although you can develop great 'knee sensitivity' by practising constantly, your knees will never be as sensitive as your hands. Therefore, they should be used with discretion and only on those areas that have previously been checked by your hands. Knees can be applied individually or together.

Keep both hands on the receiver's body so that your body weight is supported through your hands rather than through your knees. In other words, your hands must be positioned so that you can instantly remove them if necessary, to ensure the receiver's comfort and your own stability.

Using feet

Your feet can be a very useful tool for shiatsu. Although they are less sensitive than your hands, they can give a very earthy quality to a session. This is because feet spend most of their time in contact with the ground. If you intend to use your feet for shiatsu, you should walk around in bare feet as much as possible to give them an even more earthy quality.

The feet are useful tools for temporarily dispersing blocked ki in the limbs by using a rapid shaking technique, but with light and even pressure.

Offering maximum support and connection

Ensuring your recipient's physical comfort is vital to shiatsu therapy. The receiver should be supported and in a stable position. The best position is flat on the floor, face up or face down. In this position, no muscular tension is required to offset the effect of gravity.

The judicious use of cushions for comfort and support can make a great deal of difference. For example, sometimes lying face down can aggravate a weak or tender lower back, because the lumbar spine feels compressed. This can be offset by placing one or two cushions under the receiver's belly to open their lower back. When the recipient is in the face-down position, you might also want to place cushions under their feet to support their instep, especially

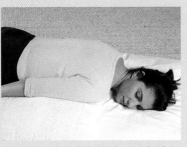

A cushion placed under the receiver's shoulder will ease neck strain.

when applying techniques to their lower legs.

Perhaps the biggest problem with the face-down position is that many people cannot get their necks into a comfortable position. If the neck is flexible enough, having the head turned to one side is the most relaxing position. People with slightly stiff necks may still be able to lie with their head turned to one side if they place their arms on the floor beyond their head. However, this does make it more difficult for the giver to access the *tsubos* around the nape of the neck and upper back. Therefore, it is better if receivers have their arms down by their sides.

When lying face up, some receivers will feel more comfortable with cushions placed behind their knees, particularly those with certain back problems. Also, those with round shoulders and/or stiff necks may be more comfortable with a

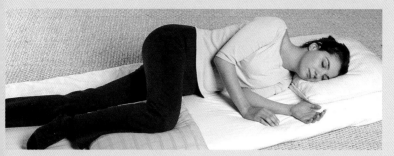

In the side position, the body should be supported at the head and knee.

cushion or pillow under their heads. Remember that some people actually prefer to lie completely flat on their backs, however, with no supporting cushions. So ask receivers what they prefer.

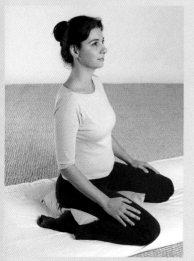

A supported kneeling position.

In the side position, you should support the head with a pillow. Also, position the legs in such a way as to prevent the receiver from rolling on to their belly.

Some people prefer to kneel, while others prefer to sit cross-legged. Kneeling can be more comfortable with a firm bolster between the legs. This will take the pressure off the thighs and insteps. Some people cannot sit cross-legged comfortably because their pelvis tilts too far back, causing lower back fatigue. Sit these people on a thick, firm cushion or a firm foam block 6–10cm deep. This will tilt their pelvis forwards and take the strain off their lower back.

Remember to initiate your movement from your *hara*, and lean rather than push. Your touch will be welcomed rather than repelled and the recipient will open up and relax rather than tensing and closing.

The rule of two-hand connection

The techniques which have the most profound effects upon the receiver's ki are those which involve having both hands in contact with the receiver's body. Your hands are your most sensitive ki imbalance detectors and ki projectors. Therefore, two hands are twice as effective as one. Two hands are even more effective if they are separated while in contact, rather than overlapping each other. As explained on page 21, in the practical application of two-hand connection, one hand will assume a more supportive role and the other a more active role.

In effect, two-hand connection is the method used to draw ki from the area beneath your support hand to the area beneath your working hand. In the process, the ki distortions in the body are smoothed out and the body/mind functions are regulated.

The object of shiatsu is to get your receiver's ki to move from their *hara* through their limbs and into their hands and feet. For this reason, the support hand should be positioned close to the centre of their body as the working hand gradually progresses away from it and thus away from the centre of the body. In other words, the hands should start close together and move apart rather than starting apart and moving together. Why? Imagine you are trying to keep track of a friend in a railway station bustling with people. It is easier to start off together and

Developing a conscious touch

To get away from a purely mechanical touch and develop the most conscious touch, you should do the following:

• With your hands apart and on the receiver's body, focus your mind on your *hara* rather than on your hands.

• Sense that your hands 'begin' in your *hara* – you can do this by

focusing on your inhalation and exhalation, as if you are breathing through your lower belly.

• Tune into the sensation that your arms and hands are 'breathing' in unison with, and as an extension of, your *hara*.

• Feel as if your 'total body' breathing includes the part of the receiver's body that lies between your hands.

maintain visual contact as your friend moves progressively further away than trying to pick her out of a crowd from a distance. Likewise, your hands can maintain ki connection with each other more easily if they start off close together.

This means we have some rules regarding two-hand connection:

• The support hand, rather than the working hand, should, where possible, be positioned close to the centre of the receiver's body.

• The working hand should move away from the support hand, not towards it.

• The support hand and the working hand should be applied with equal awareness and pressure.

Maintaining a fluent continuity of technique

The receiver will experience a feeling of integration throughout their body and mind if the giver of shiatsu can practise a fluent technique. Try to maintain contact as your hands glide from one position to the next. Making and breaking contact continuously will inhibit the receiver's ability to relax, because they will be unsure where your hand will apply shiatsu next.

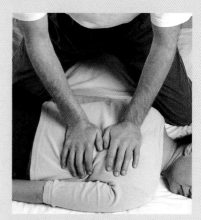

Support hand (practitioner's left hand) is stationary while the active hand (practitioner's right hand) moves.

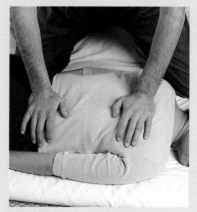

The active hand should move away from the support hand.

Do-in
Exercises

There is a system of ki-unblocking and ki-strengthening exercises known as Do-in (Japanese) or Dao-Yinn (Chinese). A shiatsu practitioner should maintain a healthy flow of ki around their own body to maximize the potential of the shiatsu techniques. Ki energy can flow from a person with a greater amount of ki to a person with less, therefore, the giver of shiatsu should practise Do-in exercises to boost and develop their ki as much as they can.

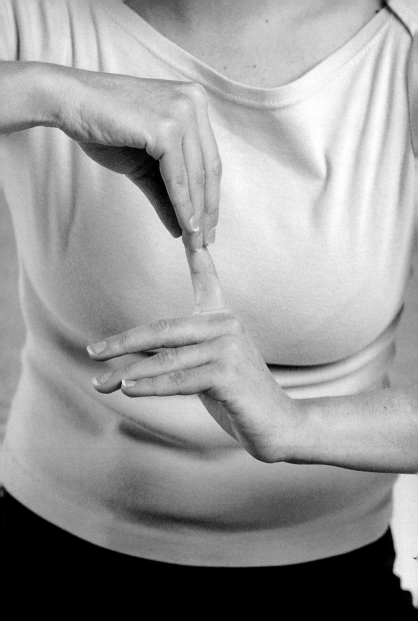

Do-in 'self-shiatsu' exercises for the hands and feet

Do-in includes a wide range of stretching, acupressure, rubbing and percussion techniques that we can apply to ourselves. Try to get into the habit of following these exercises on a regular basis and particularly before practising shiatsu.

It is outside the scope of this book to describe Do-in techniques in depth, but there is a preliminary Do-in method which can be used to keep the joints of the hands and feet supple and free of blocked ki.

For the giver of shiatsu, it is particularly helpful to keep ki flowing smoothly through the hands and feet. This is because a free flow of ki in the feet helps to keep us grounded, while a smooth ki flow through the hands ensures better touch-sensitivity during shiatsu, improving the ability to read jitsu and kyo areas. Do-in exercises for the hands also lead to a greater potential for the transmission of our healing touch.

Although Do-in techniques are traditionally performed at dawn, these exercises can be done at any convenient time.

Do-in exercises for wrist

Firstly, apply a gentle pull to your wrist joint as you exhale (making space within the joint).

Now, keeping your wrist flaccid, flap it up and down. Visualize any stiffness being dislodged and your blood flow increasing. As you continue, imagine that you are shaking out the stiffness and expelling ki stagnation; rather like water droplets from a wet cloth as you shake out the excess water.

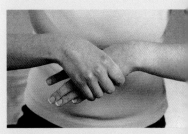

Traction to the wrist joint.

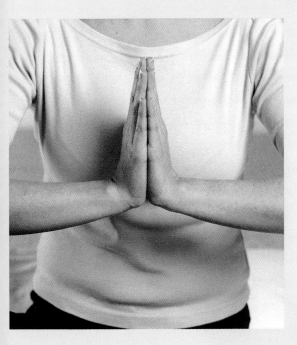

Palms together, elbows held out.

Now hold both palms together in the prayer position, with your hands held close to your chest and your elbows spread, thus extending your wrist joints. Now, move your hands down towards your waist until you feel the heels of your hands beginning to pull apart. If you practise this technique regularly, your wrist flexibility will improve, so that you will be able to bring your hands progressively further down your body, loosening your wrists and easing the flow of ki.

Imagine all restriction to these movements melting or evaporating away. You can then visualize clean oil working its way into all aspects of the wrist joint.

You can consciously influence the workings of your body if you can accept that ki will go where your mind directs it. If you clearly visualize stuck ki exiting the wrist and fresh blood and ki entering it, then that is what will happen. The more focused your mind, the better this will work.

Do-in exercises for fingers

Follow the same principles and visualizations as the wrist exercises for the following exercises.

Take hold of your index finger and apply some traction to the finger as you rotate it. Rotate it in both directions. Exhale as you apply the movement, visualizing your blood flow increasing and any waste products being expelled, along with stagnant ki.

Repeat on all fingers in turn.

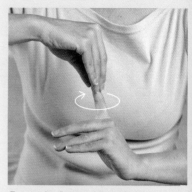

Rotate the finger while applying upwards traction.

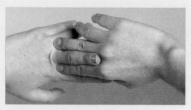

Levering finger away from palm.

Make a fork with your index and middle fingers and lever each finger of the other hand in turn, away from the palm. Exhale as you apply the movement. Imagine all restriction and stiffness melting away. Finish by flapping the hand and wrist, as for the wrist exercises.

Do-in exercises for feet

Beat the sole of your foot with your knuckles or fist for about 30 seconds. Be firm, but do not bruise yourself. Imagine you are beating the debris of ki and blood stagnation out of the foot and ankle. When you stop, imagine you can feel all the pores in the sole of your foot breathing.

Finally, stand on one leg and vigorously shake your other foot in the air. Repeat with the other foot.

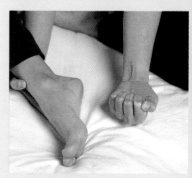

Beating the sole of the foot.

Do-in exercises for toes

Take hold of your big toe and apply some traction to it as you rotate it. Rotate it in both directions. Exhale as you apply the movement, visualizing an increased blood flow and the expulsion of waste products and stagnant ki. Repeat on all toes in turn.

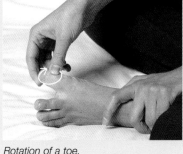

Rotation of a toe.

Gently lever each toe in turn towards the top of the foot. Exhale as you apply the movement. Imagine all restriction and stiffness melting away. Toes 3, 4 and 5 may even touch the top of the foot within a few days of practice – toes loosen up very quickly. Do not force them, however, or suffer pain.

Lever toe towards the top of the foot.

If you do these exercises when you get up in the morning, run your hands and feet under the cold tap first. Your feet especially will feel incredibly alive and warm afterwards, as blood and ki rush into them. This feeling of vitality will then quickly extend throughout your whole body. Keeping a box of pebbles under your bed to walk on immediately you get out of bed provides another good boost. It gives you a sort of instant general reflexology tonic.

Simple Sequence
in the
Prone Position

A complete sequence incorporates a range of exercises to maintain and enhance the flow of ki energy around the whole of the body. The prone position is one of the most comfortable and relaxing positions for the receiver. Remember to make the receiver comfortable before beginning and during shiatsu by following the suggestions on pages 32–33. This book is for beginners and intended as a supplement to personal or class instruction from an experienced shiatsu teacher. As outlined on page 7, you should practise these techniques only on people who are fit and well.

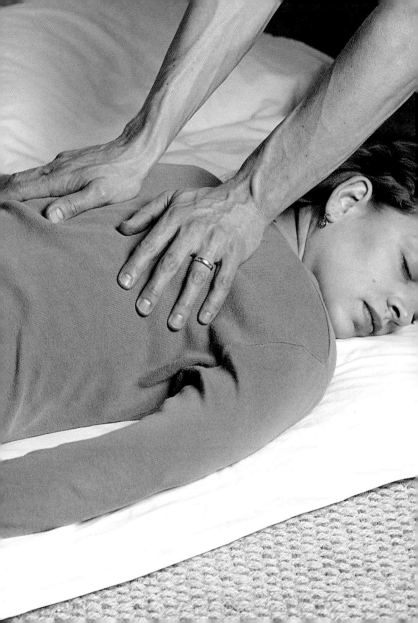

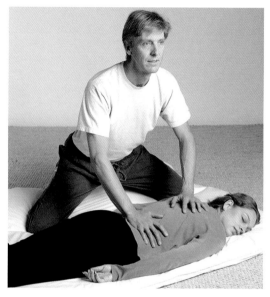

Keep your head upright, your shoulders relaxed and your hara open, following the posture guidelines on page 19.

Baby walking

Kneel next to the receiver, ensuring you spread your knees wide enough to give yourself a low centre of gravity and therefore a solid base from which to work. Keep your head up and your *hara* relaxed and open. Lean forward on to all fours, leaning your body weight through your hands and walk them randomly over the receiver's back and buttocks, just like a baby crawling. Allow gravity to determine the level of pressure rather than applying pressure through pushing. Be careful on the lower back and spinal column.

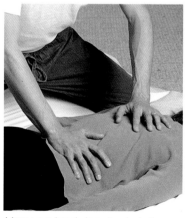

Move your hands in a steady rhythm to relax the receiver.

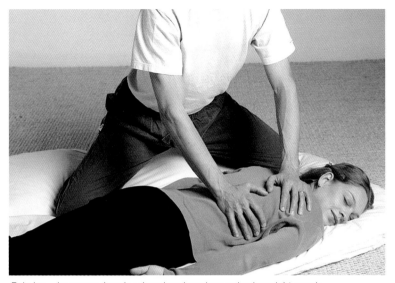

Palming – keep your hands relaxed and apply your body weight evenly.

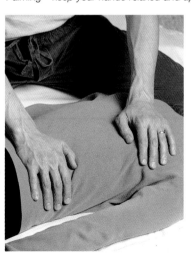

Palming

Maintain the same stance and posture as in Baby walking. Keep one hand stationary on the side of the receiver's back furthest from you, with the heel of that hand between the receiver's spine and their shoulder blade. Use your other hand to palm down the back and into the buttock, in a line just beyond the far side of the vertebral column

Remember that the stationary hand is the support hand and the hand that moves is the working hand.

Rocking

Kneel at right angles to your receiver and place both hands on their torso, on or near their waistline. If you prefer, you can place one of your hands on their sacrum or hip. Rock their body from side to side. Attune to the rhythm that seems most natural for them, which you will recognize as the rhythm which is most effortless for you to maintain. This technique is useful if the receiver is not yet fully relaxed.

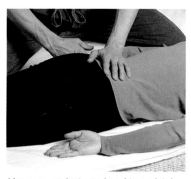

You can use just one hand to maintain a steady rocking rhythm.

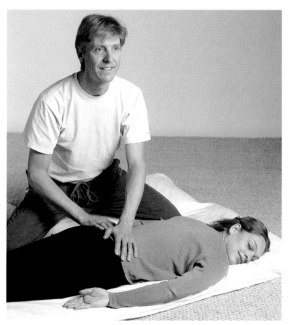

Keep your arms, shoulders and spinal column loose and soft, allowing the rocking movement to come more from your belly and hips than from your arms.

Diagonal stretch

Place one hand on the near side of the receiver's upper back, with the heel of your hand positioned close to the inside edge of their scapula (shoulder blade) and the palm of the same hand held flat against the lower half of their scapula. (Your hand should be positioned no higher than this, otherwise you will compress the receiver's neck.) Place your other hand on the buttock furthest from you so that your hands are positioned diagonally. Lean your *hara* forward towards the space between your two hands and you will feel your hands tending to splay apart. Repeat after moving your hands to the opposite shoulder blade and buttock.

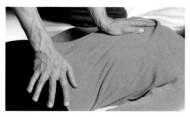

The hand positions on the shoulder blade and buttock.

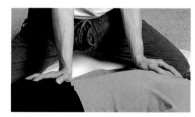

As an alternative, place both hands on the same side of the body to open one side of the back.

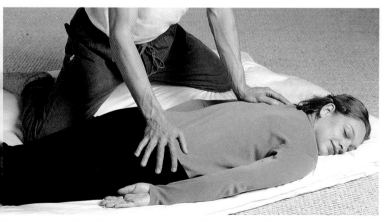

Remember not to push from the shoulder, but to lean from the hara.

Retreating cat

Move from the side of the receiver's body to just beyond their head, facing their feet. Glide both hands down the back until the heel of your hands rests on the buttocks. Gently lean your body weight forward, naturally stretching the buttocks away from the lower back, thus giving a gentle traction to the lower back. Now walk your hands from the buttocks up to the shoulder. If you like, you can walk your hands into their upper arms.

Remember not to pounce, but carefully glide your hands into the buttocks. Stretching them too suddenly or vigorously away from the lower back could weaken the ligaments of the lumbo-sacral joint and lower lumbar vertebrae.

Repeat the Retreating cat three or four times.

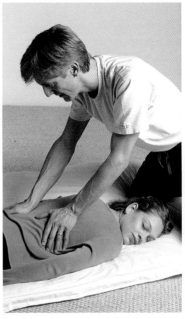

Keep your movements leisurely and consistently paced.

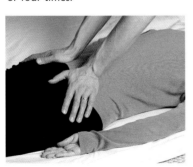

a) Your hands should be completely on the buttocks before retreating.

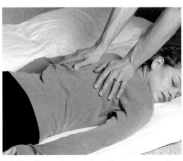

b) Don't push your hands as you walk – use your body weight.

Palm/forearm down back of legs

Kneel beside the receiver with your knee or foot adjacent to their hip and your other knee or foot adjacent to their knee or lower leg. Place your support hand on the sacrum or near-side buttock and use the other hand to palm down the back of the thigh as far as the back of the knee. Avoid leaning pressure into the back of the knee, although you can make a light connection there with your palm.

Move closer to the receiver's feet so that your support hand now rests on the lower thigh. Palm down towards the heels. Move back up so that your knee is again adjacent to the hip (without breaking contact with your hands). This time, rest one forearm against the buttock for support and use your other forearm to lean pressure into the back of the

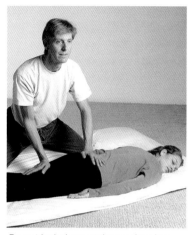

Do not look down at the receiver, but feel your way down the legs.

thigh. Finally, move your position closer to the feet so that you can again rest a support hand on the lower thigh, and repeat palming your hand towards the heels.

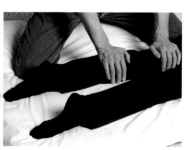

Do not lean excessive pressure into the calf, as this area is often very tender and sensitive.

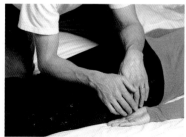

One forearm is used for support (resting on the buttock) while the other forearm applies shiatsu.

Heel to buttock

With one knee adjacent to the receiver's hip and the other knee approximately adjacent to their knee, place your support hand on the buttock and your other hand over their instep. Keeping your chest within around 30cm of the foot, bring the heel towards the buttock. At the same time, use your support hand to stretch the buttock away from the lower back.

Bringing up the foot should be performed in a slightly circular movement so that you bring the heel towards the buttock along a semi-circular or crescent-shaped path. You draw the heel away from the buttock in a similar fashion. This ensures that the technique has a smooth and fluid quality.

Some people have stiff thighs or knee joints, others are very flexible. If the heel does not easily reach the buttock, recognize the point of resistance and go no further.

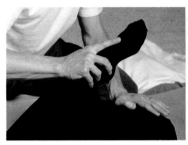

Never force or push the stretch.

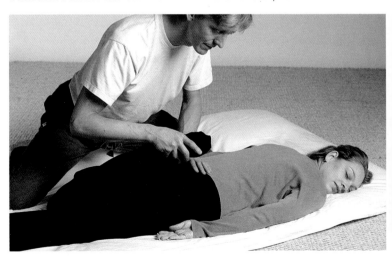

Forearms into soles

Position your thigh so that the receiver's instep comes to rest upon it. The concave shape of the angle between the ankle and the foot should fit precisely into the convex contour of your thigh, so that the foot is not dangling in mid-air. Your other knee should be resting on the back of their thigh. (If you have difficulty with this, rest your knee on the floor.) Lean your forearm into the sole of the foot, keeping your wrist fully relaxed.

The recipient's foot should be securely supported against the giver's thigh before the giver's other knee is brought on to the receiver's thigh.

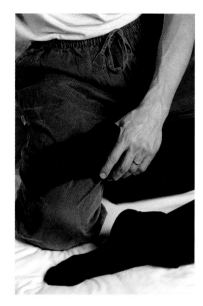

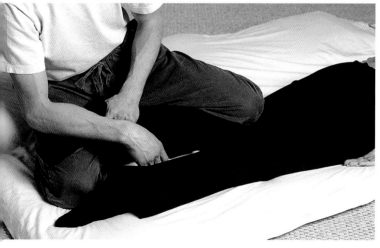

Simple Sequence
in the
Side Position

Shiatsu in the side position has certain advantages over shiatsu in other positions, as it enables full mobility of the shoulders, arms, hips and legs, plus greater movement of the torso. Also, those with back problems and women in the later stages of pregnancy often find it difficult to relax fully in any position other than the side position.

The side position requires more care for the comfort of the recipient – follow advice on page 33 for shiatsu in the side position. Also, remember to use no force in the movements other than your own body weight as this position is less stable than the prone position.

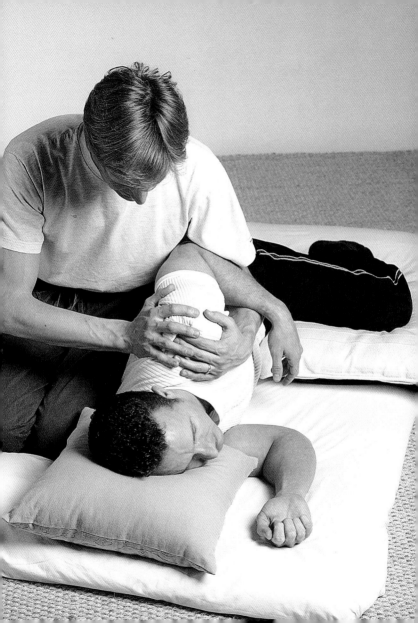

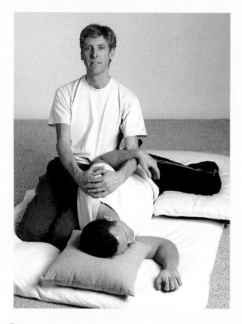

The giver should lean gently away from the shoulder without resting his body weight against the receiver.

1 Trapezius stretch

Kneel next to the receiver, facing towards their head. Kneel against their body for maximum connection, but do not push them off balance. Place their forearm over your forearm so that their arm does not drag on the floor. Clasping your hands around their shoulder, lean back using your body weight to open their neck (the upper trapezius muscle). If their head comes away from the pillow, you will know you have leaned back far too strongly, so go more gently. This technique is a great antidote to the stress-induced tension that can easily accumulate in the neck and shoulders.

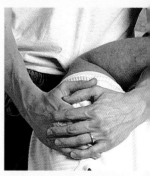

The practitioner's fingers can be overlapped or interlaced, whichever is more comfortable.

54

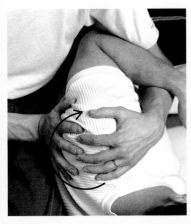

2 Shoulder girdle rotation

From the Trapezius stretch, rotate the receiver's shoulder girdle in an up, back and down direction to encourage their chest to open. Your whole body should be involved in the rotation, not just your arms.

Alternate between Trapezius stretch and Shoulder girdle rotation for one or two minutes.

The rotations must be in a up, back and down direction, or the chest will be closed by the movement.

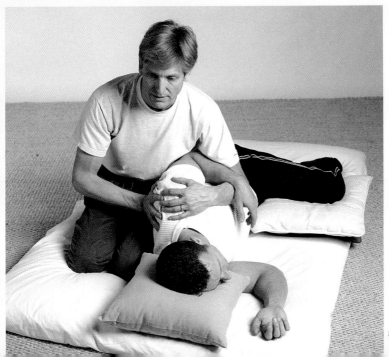

55

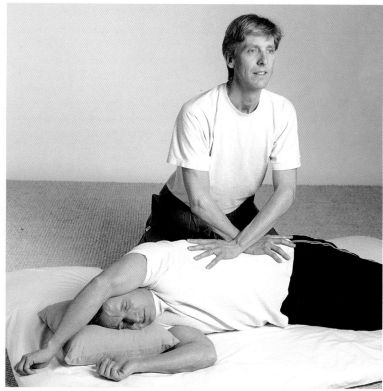

Avoid the armpit area, as this will cause discomfort to the neck and shoulder.

3 Side torso stretch

Place the receiver's hand on the floor beyond their head. If their shoulder joint lacks full mobility, you can place their arm in front of their chest. Kneel behind them mid-way between the hip and shoulder. Place their upper leg to rest just behind their lower leg. If this is not comfortable for them, leave the leg in the original position.

Cross your arms and place one hand on the hip and the other hand on the lower ribs. Lean down and open the waist area.

Arm to body stretch

Place the receiver's arm against their body. Place a cushion between the arm and the waist, to avoid stressing the elbow joint. Lean your palms into various areas along the arm and wrist. Do not lean too strongly into the corner of the shoulder, as this may cause discomfort to the neck.

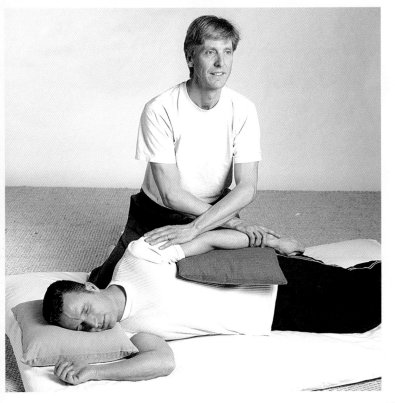

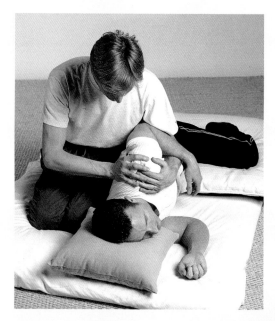

The purpose of this technique is to disperse tension in the muscles between the scapula and the vertebral column.

5 Shoulder girdle dispersing

Kneel next to the receiver, facing towards their head, as in the Shoulder girdle rotation. Place their forearm over your forearm so that their arm does not drag on the floor. Support and anchor their shoulder with one hand while you vigorously circle the heel of your other hand into and around their scapula. Try to involve your torso in the movement as much as possible, so that you minimize any tension in your arm. However, your arm will still have to work quite hard in this technique.

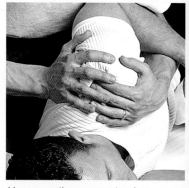

Use energetic movements when circling, or move your hand slowly and deeply as a variation.

6 Occipital opening/ neck release

Kneel close beside the receiver, but do not push them off balance. Place one hand on their forehead, without obstructing their eyes. Ideally, connect the front of their shoulder with your forearm (if it compromises your comfort, abandon this connection). Place the heel of your other hand against the nape of the neck and occiput. Explore this area with mild pressure.

This position can relieve tension headaches or tired eyes.

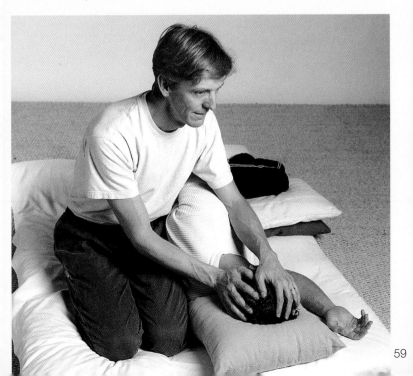

7 Knees into back

Squat behind the receiver with one hand on their shoulder and your other hand on their hip. Lean your knees against their back above the spinal column. Smoothly move your knees into various areas of the back between the buttocks and shoulder.

Avoid the tendency to round your back during this technique and keep your *hara* fully open throughout.

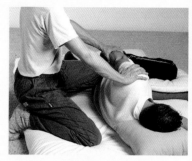

If you find it difficult using both knees together, place one knee on the floor and use one knee only on the back.

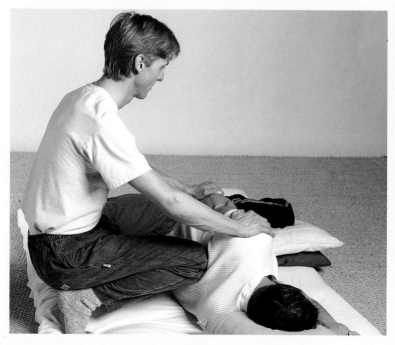

Palming the hip, thigh and leg

Position yourself behind the receiver, straddling their bottom leg. Placing one of your thumbs on top of the other, locate the centre of their buttock. Slowly lean enough pressure into this point for them to feel a definite sensation (leaning too hard will cause sharp pain). Adjust your position so that you have a support hand on their hip and can lean your other palm progressively down the outside of their thigh towards the knee.

Finish by adopting a wide kneeling stance, using both hands to palm along the lower leg.

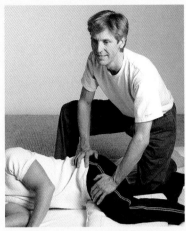

Start this position in a half kneeling stance to work on the receiver's buttocks and thighs.

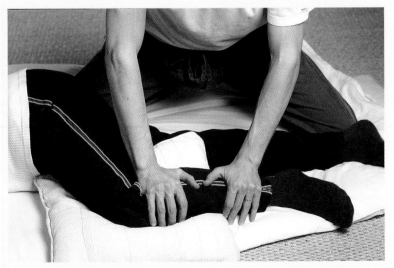

61

Useful contacts and addresses

The following organizations will be able to supply you with information and equipment on all aspects of shiatsu:

UK
The Shiatsu Society (UK)
Eastlands Court
St Peters Road
Rugby CV21 3QP
Tel: +44 (0) 1788 555051
Fax: +44 (0) 1788 555052
e-mail: admin@shiatsu.org
www.shiatsu.org
Provides a register of qualified practitioners.

The European Shiatsu School
High Bank
Lockeridge
Marlborough
Wilts SN8 4EQ.
Tel: +44 (0) 1672 513444
e-mail: info@shiatsu.org.uk
www.shiatsu.org.uk
Offers courses in London and throughout the UK and Europe.

The British School of Shiatsu-Do (Farnham)
3 Farnham Park Drive
Upper Hale
Farnham
Surrey GU9 0HS
Tel: +44 (0) 1252 724059
e-mail: registrar@bssf0shiatsu-do.co.uk
www.bssf.shiatsu-do.co.uk

London College of Shiatsu
25-7 Dalling Road
London W6 0JD
+44 (0) 20 8741 3323
www.londoncollegeofshiatsu.com

Guild of Complementary Practitioners
Liddell House
Liddell Close
Finchampstead
Berks RG40 4NS

Institute of Complementary Medicine
15 Tavern Quay
Plough Way
Surrey Quays
London SE16 1QZ

Council for Complementary and Alternative Medicine
63 Jeddo Road
London W12 9HQ

US AND CANADA
International School of Shiatsu
10 South Clinton Street
Doylestown
PA 18901
(215) 340-9918
(215) 340-9181
info@shiatsubo.com

Shiatsu School of Canada Inc.
547 College Street
Toronto
Ontario M6G 1A9
Canada
(416) 323-1818
Fax: (416) 323-1681
info@shiatsucanada.com

AUSTRALIA
Shiatsu Australia Education Centre
465 Hawthorn Foad
Caulfield Sth
VIC 3162
Australia
(03) 9528 1212
info@shiatsu-australia.com.au

Complementary Medical Association Inc.
Suite 20
1 Gladstone Road
Castle Hill
2154 NSW

USEFUL WEBSITES
www.uktherapists.com
A directory of complementary health practitioners. Includes details of training and insurance, however, these details are not validated by Uktherapists.

www.therapy4living.com
Includes general information and lists of practitioners by area for a range of complementary therapies.

Index

arm to body stretch 57
automatic nervous system (ANS) 14

baby dragon's mouth 27
baby walking 44

calming 10, 21
channels 8, 11, 12
ch'i, see ki
circular rotations 22
closed hand technique 25

diagonal stretch 46
dispersal 10, 21
dispersing claw technique 27
Do-in exercises 36, 38-41
double hand cushioning 29

elbows, using 30

feet, using 31, 41
finger techniques 26-7, 39
forearms, using 30, 49

into soles 51

grasping 22

hara 18, 19
heart disease 7
hand techniques 28-9, 30
heel to buttock technique 50
hip palming 61

index finger technique 26

jitsu 11

ki 8, 23,
blockages 11, 13, 28, 31
channels 11, 12, 13
strengthening 36
tsubos 8, 10, 13
unblocking 36
knees, using 31, 60
knuckle rolling 29
kyo 11

leg palming 61
loose finger chopping 28

occipital opening/neck release 59
open hand technique 24

palm cupping 10, 29
palming 45, 61
palm off the body technique 23
palm overlap 22
palms, as tools 20
pressure points (tsubos) 8, 10, 13
prone position techniques 44-51
pummelling 28

qi, see ki

receiver 17, 18-19
physical comfort for 32-33
retreating cat 48
rocking 46

self-shiatsu 38-41
shiatsu
aims of 11, 13
cautions 7
clothing for 6

floor area for 6
history of 4, 5
leaning principl 15, 18
meaning of 4
posture 19
relaxation response 14, 1
techniques 10, 1 18, 24-35
theory 11
tools of 6, 16
shoulder girdle dispersing 58
rotation 55
side position techniques 31, 52, 54-61
side torso stretch 56
support hand technique 21

tanden 18
three/four finger technique 26
thigh palming 61
thumbs, as tools 24-25
adjacent 25
overlap 25

varicose veins 7